Thoughts from the Heart

By

Dr. Don Loeffler, D.C

Foreword

In this book by Dr. Don, you'll find a treasure trove of valuable insights from a caring and knowledgeable doctor. His expertise shines through as he simplifies complex esoteric topics, making them accessible to everyone. His genuine dedication to helping others live more fulfilling lives is evident on every page. I wholeheartedly recommend this book—it's not just a read, but a journey guided by a compassionate expert who wants to share his wisdom for the benefit of all.

Neetu Rishi
CEO & Founder
The Success Door
Two times published author
Neeturishi.com

Table of Contents

WHAT WILL MATTER WHEN YOU'RE GONE

There will be no sunrises, no minutes, no hours, no days. All the things you've collected, whether treasures or forgotten will pass to others.

Your wealth, fame, and temporal power will shrivel to irrelevance. It will not matter what you owned or owed. Your grudges, resentments, regrets, frustrations and jealousies will finally disappear. So too, your hopes, ambitions, plans and to-do list will expire. The wins and losses that that once seemed so important will fade away. It won't matter where you lived or how. It won't matter if you're beautiful or brilliant. Even you gender and skin color will be immaterial.

So, what will matter? How will the value of your days be measured? What will matter is not what you bought, but what you built. Not what you got, but what you gave. What will matter is not your success, but your significance. What will matter is not what you learned, but what you taught. What will matter is every act of courage, compassion, integrity, or sacrifice that enriched, empowered, or encouraged others to emulate your example. What will matter is not your competence, but your character. What will matter is not how many people you know, but how many will feel a lasting loss when you're gone.

What will matter is not your memories, but the memories that live on in those who love you. What will matter most is how long you will be remembered, by whom, and for what. A life lived those matters is not of circumstance, but of choice.

We should learn to live each day to its fullest. Embrace the quiet beauty of a flower; feel the joy of a child's laughter; quietly and anonymously help someone in need; take a walk in the park.

Let go of the regrets and slights of the past. The past exists only in your mind. Living with animosity for others is like taking poison and hoping the other person dies. Bless the past and get on with the present. God grant me the serenity to accept the things I cannot change, the courage to change the things I can, and the wisdom to know the difference. That old saying is ancient, but effective and relevant.

Don't become so inured by concerns for the future that you forget to live today. Time is merely a man-made contrivance or God's way of keeping everything from happening all at once. A day to a small child may seem like an eternity while a decade to an older person may seem like a flash.

It's not who you are or what you have that will be the most important; it all pales when compared to what you are.

"We often meet our destiny on the road we take to avoid it."

"We don't see things the way they are;we see things the way we are." Talmud

TRUTH IS TRUTH AND THAT'S THAT

Nature creates life by combining molecules in a series of ever more complex wholes. If you could see your body as it really is, your perception of the nature of matter would never be the same again. 98% of all the atoms in your body were not there a year ago. Taking this one step further, if we take the diameter of a hydrogen atom (the simplest atom) to be one mm., then the diameter of the electron orbit will be about ten meters, a ratio of 1 to 10,000, and the intervening space is vacuum- a vast empty space. Far from the Ultimate Particle, the atom is actually 99.999999% empty space. If all the empty space were taken out of your body, you would be a million times smaller than the smallest grain of sand.

At the risk of wandering off into quantum theory, let me mention that our physical bodies and all matter are made up of **interacting electromagnetic fields** vibrating at tremendous frequencies which rapidly disappear when highly magnified. The laws of nature break down at the level of the very small. Resonance is a phenomenon which occurs throughout nature. So, the molecular arrangement of the physical body is really a complex network of **interwoven energy fields.** In dis-ease, these energy fields shift from equilibrium and oscillate at different and less harmonious frequencies than in health.

Nature has developed a set of Laws which are indispensable for maintaining life. When man breaks these Laws he destroys the harmony of life within himself and encounter pain and misery; that is , he punishes himself when he sets himself up above Nature. **The one who acts according to the Laws of Nature is protected by Nature, but the one who breaks the Laws must suffer Nature's displeasure.**

Our perception of reality is based on what we have learned, or rather how we have learned things. **We are influenced by early childhood experiences much more than we might think.**

The levels of order in the construction of all life are governed by unseen laws of form and substance. The subtle energies that determine form exist as repeating geometric patterns and shapes that influence the expression of systems ranging from the tiniest atom to the greatest galaxy. From the smallest to the greatest and from the greatest to the smallest, all reality is governed by the same fundamental laws. There are parallels between the reality of the microscopic realms, levels of human experience, and the macroscopic realms of the galaxies.

The human body, if one considers basic chemistry, physics, physiology, and energy patterns, can be comprehended as a teaching tool which holds within it many lessons about the true nature of Self, one's larger reality, and even the structure and nature of the universe.

Subjective reality consists of the sum total of impressions conveyed to us through our five senses and is skewed by individual beliefs, prejudices, and fears. **Objective reality** is the **way things really are**. The world that we perceive with our five senses and the true nature of reality are actually two completely different things. It is in understanding this paradox that we can get a firm handle on how the body really works and make some serious headway into the wellness and longevity quandary.

It is very difficult to "unlearn" something that we have been programmed to believe. Growth in wisdom and awareness can be difficult and sometimes painful. It is much easier to accept everything like good little sheep than to question things that don't add up. Many times, it takes a complete generation to discard antiquated concepts or belief systems. Fifty years ago, weight training was thought to be for narcissistic egomaniacs. Nowadays, a large percentage of the population works out. Similar shifts in diet, aerobic (and anaerobic) exercise, and chiropractic have gradually replaced obsolete public perceptions to become more accepted as an integral part of health and longevity.

Both aphorisms: **"Ignorance is bliss"** and **"What you don't know can't hurt you"** are miserably wrong. Knowledge and wisdom are the keys to achieving your health goals. Many studies have shown that educated people live longer. However, there is a very important difference between knowledge and wisdom. **Knowledge void of wisdom can be a very dangerous and self-destructive thing.**

Age has many virtues; and wisdom, gained from experience, is high among them. I'm attempting in this publication, to share important highlights from many diverse sources. No doubt, this compilation of information will be constantly revised as more research is available.

"Ignorance is merely the lack of knowledge."

"The absence of evidence does not mean the evidence of absence."

"People think and act based on their own internal representation of the world, not on the world itself."

THE WELLNESS MODEL

We are taught to believe that diagnosing and treating specific diseases or illnesses is "Health Care". Nothing could be further from the truth.

Contrary to popular belief, it is possible to eliminate or ameliorate an illness or degenerative condition without specifically treating it. In the absence of conditions that will feed a disease, wellness is promoted. This is not a common idea for the average American who thinks that they are "well" as long as they have not been diagnosed with a "condition". The average person, by means of the unhealthy lifestyle they lead, is in the process of creating dis-ease*, for which a specific illness is just one of the end stages of the process. By the time a cancer manifests in that individual's body, he could have been damaging himself for twenty or thirty years. By the time he has a heart attack or stroke, he might have been living an unhealthy lifestyle for decades.

If you can see the logic behind these concepts, then I have a question for you. Why wait to end up with the unwelcome or unpleasant consequences of a disease (or dis-ease) process that develops because you have been making unwise choices, when you have the potential to prevent or reverse these degenerative processes in the first place?

Try not to end up like the old guy who once said to me: "If I knew I was going to live this long, I'd have taken better care of myself."

The term "dis-ease" refers to a state of poor health and nonspecific degeneration that may or may not include specific disease conditions such as cancer, heart disease, diabetes, arthritis, etc.

"We live in a society that takes sickness and disease for granted and looks upon high level wellness as lucky or fortuitous."

A NEW WAY TO THINK ABOUT RULES TO LIVE BY

Moral codes that seek to regulate human behavior have been with us not only since the dawn of civilization but also among our precivilized, and highly social, hunter-gatherer ancestors.

The Golden Rule

The most admired standard of behavior in the West is the Golden Rule. Its formulation in the first-century Gospel of St. Mathew is: "Do unto others as you would have them do unto you." Almost no one follows it consistently.

The Silver Rule

The Silver Rule is different. "Do not do unto others what you would not have them do unto you." This rule is different from the Golden Rule in that a wide discrepancy exists in what people like done to them. One could also argue that some individuals are quite particular about what they do not want done to them, Thus, the circular logic continues.

The Brazen Rule

"Repay kindness with kindness," said Confucious describing relations between individuals, "but evil with justice." This might be called the Bronze or Brazen Rule: "Do unto others as they do unto you." In actual human (and chimpanzee) behavior it's a familiar standard.

The Iron Rule...and others

Of baser coinage is the Iron Rule: "Do unto others before they do it unto you." It's sometimes formulated as: "He who has the gold makes the rules." This rule demonstrates not only rejection, but contempt for the Golden Rule. This is the secret maxim of many, if they can get away with it, and often the unspoken precept of the powerful.

Mixed Rules

Finally, I should mention two mixed rules, found throughout the human species world (and elsewhere). They explain a great deal. One is: "Suck up to those above you and intimidate those below." It's really the Golden Rule for superiors, the Iron Rule for inferiors. We'll call this the Tin Rule. The other common rule is: "Give precedence in all things to close relatives, and do as you like to all others." –The Golden Rule for relatives, the Iron Rule for   others. This Nepotism Rule is known to evolutionary biologists as "Kin Selection."

The Prisoner's Dilemma is a simple game which tests integrity, altruism and loyalty between two friends. Being charged with a crime, before they can collaborate on their story, they are individually interrogated and offered a chance to plead guilty to the offense. If they both plead innocents, the authorities would be hard pressed to prove guilt and the sentences would be light (if any). If they both plead guilty, the sentence would be moderate for both friends. If one pleads innocent and the other pleads guilty, the first friend would receive the maximum sentence while the second would receive a much lighter sentence. Therein lies the dilemma.

The Prisoner's Dilemma is a very simple game. Real life is considerably more complex. But its central lessons are substantial. Be consistent in who you are. Forgive your enemy if he forgives you. Treat everyone the same until given a good reason not to. However difficult it is to reconcile altruistic motives with the necessities of defense against those with less lofty rules of conduct, remain true to your own ideals. Who was it that once said: "Whatsoever you do unto the least of us, you do unto me"? What would the world be like if more of us, individuals as well as nations, lived by these rules?

"The conventional serves to protect us from the painful job of thinking."
John Kenneth Galbraith

BECOME A FRINGE-DWELLER

Many of us search for a special meaning in life and are disappointed when it never seems to happen. We fail to realize that specialness is a construct of the ego and that we can never have enough of what we don't really want. This imagined specialness becomes a restriction from which we can never escape, so long as we give it our power. If you feel entitled, or that God has a special purpose for your life, think again. Truth be told, God has a special purpose for everybody's life. We become slaves to our own ego and don't realize what freedom there is in not needing to be overtly special.

There is much specialness to be found in the everyday world. The uniqueness of each human interaction and experience offers diverse ways to fulfill whatever intrinsic need we might have for recognition of specialness.

The term "fringe-dweller" was coined by Stuarte Wilde to define free thinkers. Mainstream thinking employs a follow-the-herd mentality. Unfortunately, much of the time the herd is leading you right over the cliff. As laughable as it may seem, a good rule-of-thumb in making important decisions regarding your long-term health and taking wellness to the next level is to take a good look at what everybody else is doing, and do the exact opposite. That is, unless you feel comfort and security in living with chronic health issues and taking drugs for most of your adult life, most of which are meant to counteract the side effects of your original drugs. Meanwhile your liver and kidneys are overstressed detoxifying all the poisons.

Fringe-dwellers are not afraid to think outside of the box. In terms of medical and scientific advances, the most profound leaps in understanding profound concepts and in technological advances have come from the ideas of fringe dwellers. It is when someone has the courage and insight to see what others have seen and to think what no one else has thought, that true advancement can transpire. It is in doing the same things and thinking the same thoughts over and over again, expecting different results, that insanity emerges. While there may be a modicum of security and safety in becoming creatures of habit, when our habits are self-destructive, we are unable to achieve our potential. Discover the freedom of no longer being shackled by conventional wisdom, which is usually only partially correct in its assumptions. See what others see, but with new eyes. The results may be startling. But, be careful what you ask for, you might get it. Sometimes, we need to stray from the beaten path with the implicit trust that we will be safe. This reality is full of mysteries. We neither need to, nor can we solve them all. We just need to be open to the possibilities.

WHAT IF YOU SLEPT

And what if in your sleep you dreamed
And what if in your dream you went to heaven
And there plucked a strange and beautiful flower
And what if when you awoke
You had that flower In your hand
Ah, what then?
Samuel Taylor Coleridge

LIFE IS KINDA LIKE THAT

What if we sleepwalk through life on automatic pilot, letting others influence our perceptions and thoughts, our prejudices and predispositions, our hopes and fears, letting others make decisions that impact our health and wellness, relinquishing the right to claim our own identity and falling into the abyss of mediocrity, physically as well as spiritually? Ah, what then?

What if the body doesn't really make mistakes, but we do in the lifestyle decisions we make and merely blame our health problems on bad luck or genetics or anything else we can think of, anything but ourselves? Ah what then?

What if the quick-fix mentality foisted on us through the constant bombardments of drug commercials and advertisements is really a ploy by the multi-billion-dollar pharmaceutical corporations to generate gargantuan profits without concern for the health or well-being of their clientele or the side-effects that indiscriminate drug use effectuates?

Ah, what then?

What if we collectively decided that enough is enough and chose to be responsible for our own health, realizing that the choices we make are more accountable for the present and future state of our health than any mass-marketed pharmaceutical conspiracy and decided that we no longer choose to be lemmings being led off the side of a cliff to our own demise? Ah what then?

I'M NOT SPECIAL

As we meander through life, we oftentimes stumble over some uncomfortable truths, pick ourselves up, dust ourselves off, and proceed as if nothing had happened.

We live on a minor planet orbiting an ordinary star, one of a hundred billion stars making up the Milky Way galaxy. Beyond the Milky Way, powerful telescopes can see a hundred billion other galaxies spread throughout space.

Our universe began approximately 13 1/2 billion years ago. Planet earth formed roughly 9 billion years later. The first primitive life showed up about 4 billion years ago. The first modern man allegedly evolved much later (somewhere between 2,000 and 2-4 million years ago depending on who you talk to). Over 99% of the species that have ever inhabited earth are now extinct. Why do we think that we are so special? The odds are greatly in the favor of mankind enjoying a brief reign as "king of the world" and then fading into oblivion. Global warming may play a significant role in that outcome. How comforting is that? Do you think it matters a twit how important you are or how much money you make? If you want to be buried with your money, we'll write you a check.

It is with self-deception that we deprive ourselves of an esoteric plethora of hidden knowledge, wisdom, and spiritual growth. Some people choose to be in control of a self-limiting existence, while others have the courage to take the plunge into the unknown and enigmatic worlds. The more you realize how little you know, the more open your mind can be. Humans possess two fundamental motivations: fear and desire. Fear of the unknown causes us to cling tenaciously to the dogmas that define superficial existence. Desires for materialistic gains circumvent us from of seeking more valuable insights into the deeper mysteries of life that are much more important than anything mundane.

There may come a time in your life when you realize that you are not special. With that realization emerges a liberation that frees you to experience life for what it truly is. We tend to become unwitting slaves to our egos and relate to one another in roles rather than as souls. Robbing the ego of its power to control you is as easy as being yourself and genuinely enjoying the miracles of life and really getting its true meaning.

"No Religion has a Monopoly on God's Truth"
Clerics Assert

THE PITFALLS OF NEW AGE SPIRITUALITY

1. **Narcissism:** There's a thin line between narcissism and "following your bliss". Without some degree of sacrifice for the greater good, self-discovery eventually leads to plain old self-indulgence. A recent research study showed a strong relationship between heart disease and the propensity of the individual to liberally sprinkle their conversation with such words as I, me and mine, which reflect self-centeredness.

2. **Superficiality:** 21st-Century Spirituality is often culpable of espousing superficial and affable answers to life's complexity and pain. Spirituality must not be used to shield ourselves from the rough-and-tumble of real life. Any world-view that suggests that thinking positively always protects you from harm, or that there is something wrong with you if you suffer or fail, or that healing isn't often difficult and complex, is offering empty promises.

3. **The Never-Ending Process of Self-Improvement:** You can become so obsessed with your own self-

improvement-your story, your victimization, your faults, your fears, your regrets- that instead of becoming free, you end up caught in an endless loop. This myopic focus on the self often leads to social apathy and withdrawal. Nobody is perfect. Accept yourself for who you are, warts and all, and go from there.

4. **Instant Transformation:** Dear God, Please give me patience and give it to me right now. Just as the never-ending process of self-examination seduces some people, others are disappointed when they don't achieve inner peace after reading a book or taking a workshop. Spiritual awakening takes patience, hard work, and the grace of God.

5. **Desire for Magic:** Don't throw common sense out the window in the search for God. The need to rely on all-powerful teachers, angelic visitations, spirit guides and other esoteric assistance can obscure the ordinary magic of everyday life. There is much to be learned from watching small children or animals play.

6. **Grandiosity:** If you find yourself becoming unbearably profound, feeling that you are somehow special and destined for greatness, perhaps you are

suffering from grandiosity. Your message will be much more readily accepted if you are coming from a place of humility and concern for others. People don't care how much you know until they know how much you care.

7. **Romanticizing Indigenous Cultures:** There exists a kind of reverse prejudice in our politically correct times that just because some teaching is from another culture or a far away land, especially an indigenous culture or territory, that it is somehow more enlightening, spiritual, or wise. There is a direct relationship between how far one must travel and the profoundness of the teachings, or so we think.

8. **The Inner-Child Tantrum:** When praying, remember that God always answers our prayers. Be aware, however, that frequently the answer is "no". It is good and just to know what you want, respect your own needs, and honestly ask for what you feel you deserve. But is also important to know when to acquiesce to insights higher than your own.

9. **Ripping Off the Traditions:** Many modern seekers plunder the ritual

trappings of a tradition with little respect for the depth behind them. This behavior trivializes stalwart and elegant systems of spiritual growth that often demand years of study. There is a difference between carefully creating a spiritual path that includes genuine practices from a variety of legitimate traditions and flitting from flower to flower like a drunken honeybee,

10. **The Guru Trip:** Perhaps the most baffling and trying aspect of 21st-Centruy Spirituality is the disparity between spiritual teachings and the behavior of some teachers. Men, women, Eastern, Western, fundamentalist, New Age, modern, or indigenous- few escape the temptation to abuse power. Some do so blatantly. Things to be wary of: extravagant claims of enlightenment or healing powers, excessive commercialism that betrays the deeper spiritual message, and the blind devotion of followers to charlatans.

"All truth passes through three stages first it is ridiculed second it is violently opposed third it is accepted as being self-evident"
Arthur Schopenhauer

FOUR STAGES OF LEARNING

The acquisition of knowledge and wisdom tend to pass through four distinct phases on the way to intellectual and emotional assimilation. They can be road-blocked at any phase as the ego's defense mechanisms can be quite persistent. The four stages of learning that we pass through are Unconscious Incompetence, Conscious Incompetence, Conscious Competence, and Unconscious Competence.

1. **Unconscious Incompetence:** This is the stage where you don't know what you don't know. You tend to violently resist any concepts or ideas that contradict the paradigm that you have constructed around yourself. The ego is at its' arrogant best.

2. **Conscious Incompetence:** This is where you begin to realize there is something that you don't know. Sometimes this phase is like a gradual awakening from a deep sleep.

3. **Conscious Competence:** This is where you realize that there are things that you don't know, but you have to remind yourself as old habits die hard. Truth can't be unlearned, but it can be ignored, at least for a while.

4. **Unconscious Competence:** This where implementation becomes second nature. You subconsciously and automatically incorporate your newfound wisdom into your perceptions, interpretations and lifestyle.

"It ain't what you don't know that gets you into trouble; it's what you know for sure that just ain't so."
      Mark Twain

"The main difference between truth and fiction is that fiction has to make sense."

"Half the truth is often a great lie."
      Benjamin Franklin

SCIENCE-RELIGION-PHILOSOPHY
HOW THEY FORM OUR BELIEFS

SCIENCE: The observation, identification, description, experimental investigation, and theoretical explanation of phenomena.
RELIGION: Belief in and reverence for a supernatural power or powers, regarded as creator and governor of the universe.
PHILOSOPHY: The investigation of causes and laws underlying reality.

As the casual observer can clearly see, science, religion and philosophy are not mutually exclusive. There is substantial overlap in the study and application of each. The beauty and complexity of nature must have organization and intelligence behind it. The exact set of circumstances necessary for life to begin and evolve is beyond chance. No intelligent person will argue with that.

How do science, religion, and philosophy influence our paradigm?

The conceptual framework that permits the explanation and investigation of the existence we call life or our world-view paradigm tends to wrap itself up in a neat little cocoon from which it is very difficult to escape. It is similar to the spider web that envelopes the helpless insect. The more it struggles, the tighter the restriction. Looking at reality through a "new set of eyes" takes a modicum of courage. Tony Robbins once said that for someone to change, the pain of not changing must become greater than the pain of changing. It may take hardship, struggle, and even catastrophe to implement an awakening. But those who search for truth in a meaningful and sincere way are often rewarded with esoteric knowledge and wisdom that far surpasses their expectations. Sometimes that can be a very lonely place. Be careful what you ask for. The answers can be disconcerting.

Paradigms are never true or false. A paradigm is the arena in which our personal interpretations are played out. It is these interpretations that are true or not true. We must remember, just because we believe something to be true, doesn't make it so. Our personal paradigm is basically formed long before we reach the age of reason and discernment. Science's influence is felt through influences of everyday phenomena that we inherently take for granted. Religion's influence is felt in our intrinsic search for a higher meaning in life. The influence of philosophy is felt through our need for explanations (as long as they fit neatly within our paradigm-and there lies the conundrum).

"I am going to do today what other people are not willing to do, so I can do tomorrow what other people cannot."

Jerry Rice

Moods: You generate them yourself and then find your excuse for having them.

SENSE OR NO SENSE?

Common sense is neither common nor is it sense. It is defined as having or exhibiting native good judgment.

Nonsense is that which does not fit into the prearranged patterns that we have envisioned for our personal realities. What we take for sensible is nothing but our personal camouflage of the underlying reality. The only way to escape from the dogmas that enslave us is to venture from established lines of thought. We must venture into the point of view that nonsense may not be nonsense at all. In fact, viewed through new eyes it might become perfectly obvious. Once we admit to ourselves that the emperor has no clothes, we begin to realize that nonsense from an old point of reference can make perfect sense from a new place of reference. We once believed that the earth was flat. In fact, the Flat Earth Society still has valid arguments why the earth really is flat. Truth be told, just about any argument can seem valid, depending on the underlying premises that form its foundation. There is a certain faction that truly believes the holocaust never happened. We have been taught to believe that bacteria and viruses are the cause of ill health and disease. The consequences have produced more drugs and treatments, but with failing results. The billions spent on medical research for diseases such as cancer, heart disease, and diabetes have produced only limited resolutions, with the primary benefit being early detection.

Reality is what we take to be true.
What we take to be true is based upon what we believe.
What we believe is based upon our perceptions.
What we perceive depends upon what we look for.
What we look for depends upon what we are familiar with.
What we are familiar with depends upon what we have seen in the past.
What if our past experiences began with false premises?
Would our current reality be then laden with falsehoods?
Would we cling tenaciously to old paradigms that have proven ineffective?

We are constantly inundated with a media blitz of symptom-chasing medications. If we have any hopes of reversing the trend of chronic diseases that is engulfing our nation, we must learn to look in unpopular places for answers to fundamental questions. Dare to see what others have seen and think what no one else has thought. We are currently laden with false premises and ineffective paradigms.

SETH SPEAKS

There are higher meanings to life that transcend the mundane. How's that for a shocker? There's more to life than chasing little green pieces of paper. Each of us lives behind a wall, beyond which lies the infinite potential of the unknown.

If you have a limited concept of the nature of reality, then your ego will do its best to keep you in the small enclosed area of your accepted paradigm. If, on the other hand, your intuition and creative instincts are allowed freedom, they will communicate knowledge of greater dimensions to this most physically oriented portion of your personality.

We perceive our reality within very limited parameters. Our five senses detect a very restricted slice of the total picture. With the advent of quantum physics, new ways of looking at the world emerged. The metamorphosis of this new and unique science required intuitive knowledge, which is far superior to any other kind. Albert Einstein was a master of thinking outside the box.

Events in your life are not necessarily things that "happen" to you. In many cases, they are materialized experiences formed by you according to your beliefs and expectations. It should be obvious that you draw to yourself those circumstances upon which you concentrate your attention. The thoughts in which you are the most strongly emotionally invested are formed into physical reality by very definite methods and through laws quite valid, though they may not be presently understood. If you vividly concern yourself with the injustices, you feel have been done you, then you will attract more such experiences. If you play the role of victim or martyr, then you will attract events that feed that role. He who hates an evil merely creates another one. If you release yourself from animosity, then you automatically release yourself from any such relationships in the future- or any experiences that are based on enmity. Each of us has an intuitive sense of our life's purpose, but we need to get out of our own way. Suffering is not good for the soul unless it teaches you to stop suffering. Remember, a soul is not something that you have. It is what you are and is itself the most highly energized and potent consciousness in this or any other universe.

*"There is one great good in life-wisdom
and one great evil-ignorance."*

          Socrates

HOW TO LIVE A HAPPY, HEALTHY AND MEANINGFUL LIFE

Exercise Your Mind

The second component of a happy, healthy and meaningful life is a searching and evolving mind. Become aware of the infinite possibilities to learn of the miracles of nature, science, history, art, etc. Challenge your mind at every opportunity to learn new things and constantly seek to broaden your horizons. Life's experiences offer many chances to learn and evolve. Learn from your experiences and some of life's more difficult lessons will be less likely to be repeated over and over again.

Honor Your Spirit

The third component of a fulfilling and meaningful life lies in honoring your spirit. Awaken to the miracle that is life and honor the process of your own spiritual evolution. Take the time and put forth the effort to look beyond the illusion that is mundane life and embark on the only journey that results in fulfillment and real meaning to your existence.

Keys to Fulfillment

1. Certainty

We need routine and sameness to our lives. We need a certain amount of control and comfort as we move toward pleasure and away from pain.

2. Uncertainty

We also need a dose of uncertainty in the form of variety and surprise to keep life interesting. Everyone must find their own balance between too much and not enough uncertainty.

3. Significance

Everyone must feel a uniqueness or a specialness to those around them. Sometimes this is achieved through default where an individual elevates himself through default by tearing others down. True significance, however, is realized with the understanding that we all are unique and special in our own way and no one is exactly like you.

4. Connection

No man is an island. We all need to connect with members of our own species. We can also connect with Nature or through mutual problems such as the tragedy of 9-11. Being part of a group and connecting with others is vital in reaching fulfillment.

5. Personal Growth

We must all continue to grow and evolve or life loses its meaning. Personal growth is what life is all about. Growth can take many forms. There are many useful books and tapes by such authors as Deepak Chopra, Wayne Dyer, Stuart Wilde, Tony Robbins, Jerry Stocking, Dick Sutphen, Marianne Williamson and many others that can guide us on this journey. Sometimes quiet introspection can be more valuable than any number of counseling sessions. Some of the most profound insights come in the silent space between our thoughts.

6. Contribute beyond yourself.

We all have an innate need to feel as if we're a part of something bigger than ourselves. We need to contribute to the betterment of mankind through some type of selfless service without the expectation of reward and as anonymously as possible.

Emotional pain is felt when one or more of these criteria is not being met. No matter how much money we have, no matter how much material security we possess, the ego will always want more and will never be satisfied.

"The only true fulfillment is found in respecting your body, exercising your mind, and honoring your spirit."

"We do not see things as they are. we see things as we are."

"When you change the way, you look at things the things you look at change."

"No tree has branches so foolish as to fight amongst themselves."

Respect Your Body

In life we have two homes. One of these homes (the family home) is where we keep our stuff while we go out and accumulate more stuff. Our other home (our personal home) is where our spirit resides. Neither of these homes is who we really are. Both are transitory. The first home we can easily leave for a bigger and better one. The second home is where we spend an entire lifetime. Much like an automobile, we make choices regarding how we care for this home. However, with an automobile, when something goes wrong, we can open it up, take out the bad piece and put in a new one. We are not that fortunate with the physical body. The condition of this home is mainly contingent on choices that we make over the course of its existence. Many of the choices that we make earlier in life affect us as we get older. The level of our health and fitness in our fifties and sixties is largely determined by lifestyles decisions we make in our thirties and forties.

"When you open your heart, you will experience not learned intelligence rather innate intelligence."

DENIAL'S NOT A RIVER
IN EGYPT

Each individual interprets his/her own intrinsic perception of life and its vicissitudes according to four distinct parameters: what they know, what they want, what they believe, and what they feel. It's like four trains coming together in a collision course. When these four verisimilitudes collide, you get left with the unconfusing, unobfuscated, unadulterated and uncomplicated truth, as they see it. Therein lays the rub. It's a wonder society can even function, given so many different truths floating around like butterflies dancing in the wind.

We make decisions based on emotions dating back 100 million years from the primitive limbic system and justify these decisions in our rational, cortical mind which dates back a mere 4 million years.

What is unfortunate for the vast majority of the population is that believing something to be true or not true does not really make it so. An individual who is uncomfortable with the real truth will tend to lapse into denial. This line of thinking may not pose a significant threat to their well-being if it does not involve issues of health and dis-ease. Here we tread on dangerous grounds.

Unfettered scientific research and achievements

routinely intrude on every aspect of human and natural life. The wall between fiction and reality has become almost indistinguishable. Our technical and scientific capabilities have brought the world to a turning point, one in which accomplishments and innovations in the health care field are at odds with the old-fashioned natural processes of the inner wisdom of the human body.

Science has trespassed on nature's venue; it has forgotten what was authentic and has transgressed upon nature's wisdom. We have assumed that discovering how to manipulate nature has moved us forward, when the exact opposite may be true.

Science devoid of philosophy and morality can be a very dangerous thing. When the bottom line becomes more important than intellectual honesty, an unpredictable can of worms is opened and we may unwittingly be crushed by the bulldozer of "progress".

The public has come to expect miracles, but has little faith in those entrusted to produce them, a logical skepticism given the economic incentives of the scientific and pharmaceutical communities. We have acquired more knowledge in the past decade than in the previous two centuries and we may not be spiritually and ethically advanced enough to properly utilize this new knowledge; for without wisdom, knowledge can be a very dangerous thing.

Developing a healthy doctor-patient relationship creates a sacred space that allows trust and a willingness to work together to find the best solution to the patient's problems, problems that are most efficiently resolved when the doctor is unfettered by pharmaceutical conflicts of interest.

Questions of pharmaceutical efficacy are often bolstered by accurate information taken wildly out of context, wielded selectively, and supported by "experts" with compelling arguments.

Even as scientists around the world race to unlock the intricacies of the human genome, they are getting dangerously close to creating new life forms, much like a Frankenstein, but less predictable. We may unleash our own demise through viral manipulations which may inevitably present the biggest single threat to man's continued dominance on this planet. We may be unable to put the genie back in the bottle.

The scientists who are reconstructing extinct viruses may very well be remembered as the most irresponsible scientists in the history of the world. They may inadvertently or otherwise be playing God without the wisdom or knowledge to accurately predict with certainty the ramifications of their actions. They may get us all before global warming has a chance. This behavior is a classic example of living in denial and putting personal agendas ahead of the public welfare.

"When one is looking for answers it is often helpful to know what questions to ask."

WHAT CONSTITUTES RESEARCH FRAUD?

It is simply no longer possible to believe much of the clinical research that is published, or to rely on the judgment of trusted physicians or authoritative medical guidelines. I take no pleasure in this conclusion, which I reached slowly and reluctantly over my two decades as an editor of The New England Journal of Medicine.

-Marcin Angell, New York Review of Books

January 15, 2009

Three Major catalysts for Research Fraud
1. Career pressure- the researcher feels compelled or obligated to reach certain predetermined conclusions.
2. The researcher thinks he knows how the experiments are supposed to turn out. He often, however, also knows what the outcome would be if he were to exhibit intellectual honesty.
3. The research is performed under circumstances that are not precisely reproducible.

Serious conflict of interest is rife in research medicine, a fact well documented to exist even at its highest levels in universities, regulatory agencies, and prestigious medical journals.

Scientific fraud is almost always a transgression against the methods of scientific research, not purposely against the body of knowledge. What data is interpreted is generally above reproach; how it is interpreted is where the wiggle-room exists. This is nowhere more evident than in the biomedical area where multimillion dollar research grants are contingent on research findings.

Scientific research and experimentation is usually chaotic; you don't know what's going on; you cannot usually understand what the data means; but in the end you draw your own conclusions and then, with hindsight, you write it up as one clear and certain step after another. This is a kind of hypocrisy, but one that is so deeply embedded in the way that scientific research is conducted that it is not even considered it a misrepresentation. Every scientific paper is written as if the particular investigation it describes were a triumphant progression from one truth to the next. The twin pillars of scientific research- the reward system and the authority structure are deeply flawed and must be eliminated before intellectual honesty can become the bastion for unbiased, unfettered scientific insight that is free from underlying economic and self-aggrandizement agendas.

Truth is an emotional construct. People seldom make rational decisions. They make emotional decisions and justify them through rational thought. Under such circumstances, no wonder people are confused; they just don't know who or what to believe. This is the primary reason why people choose to go down with the ship when faced with a critical health issue; they would rather face a certain familiar demise than wander from their comfort zone.

People who sail planes into skyscrapers literally believe stories that are metaphors. There are currently about 40 wars being fought in the world today that are justified through stories that are based on what is known, wanted, believed, and felt. Each side has its own rationalization for killing and destroying the enemy and they truly believe that their God is better and wiser and more powerful than the other guy's God. Who can argue with that?

Sigmund Freud named the fear of death as quite probably the major factor that drives humans to create and defend the concept of gods and religion.

"Knowing that we do not know- and being clear about it- is not a weakness; it's a virtue, a sign of strength and character."

"If the mind were simple enough that we could understand it, our minds would be so simple that we could not understand anything."

RULES FOR BEING HUMAN

1. **YOU WILL RECEIVE A BODY**- You may like it or hate it, but it will be yours for an entire lifetime.

2. **YOU WILL LEARN LESSONS**- You are enrolled in a full-time school called life. Each day you will have the opportunity to learn lessons. You may or may not recognize the value of a particular lesson. However, it will be there for your benefit.

3. **THERE ARE NO MISTAKES, ONLY LESSONS**- Growth is a process of trial and error. Failure is just as much a part of the process as success. Success and failure are arbitrary and subjective.

4. **A LESSON IS REPEATED UNTIL LEARNED**- A specific lesson will be presented to you in various forms until you have learned it. When you have learned it, you can then go on to the next lesson.

5. **LEARNING LESSONS DOES NOT END**- There is no part of life that does not contain its lessons. If you are alive, there are lessons to be learned.

6. **"THERE" IS NO BETTER THAN "HERE"**- When your "there" has become a "here", you will simply obtain another "there" that will, again, look better than

"here". You can never get enough of what you don't really want.

7. **OTHERS ARE MERELY MIRRORS OF YOU**- You cannot love or hate something about another person unless it reflects to you something you love or hate about yourself.

8. **WHAT YOU MAKE OF YOUR LIFE IS UP TO YOU**- You have everything you need to be exactly whom and what you need to be. What you do with your opportunities is up to you.

9. **YOUR ANSWERS LIE INSIDE YOU**- When we stop looking to outside sources for answers to our innermost questions, we can then realize that the answers that we so desperately seek are already inside us. All you need to do is look, listen and trust. The deepest insights and intuitions come through in the silent space between our thoughts.

10. **YOU WILL FORGET ALL THIS!**

"Discover in all things that which shines and is beyond corruption."

THE MIND OF MAN

The mind of man does not exist in time, does not occupy space, and involves, so far as anyone knows, no energy transformations. But the nervous system, through which the mind of man operates, does exist in time, does occupy space, and does require energy transformations. Admittedly, this is a mystery. How can a non-material entity such as the mind actually influence the organic nervous system? YET, WE KNOW THAT IT DOES! An idea is just as valid a stimulus to the nervous system as a kick in the teeth. Thoughts are things and deserve their rightful place in the scheme of medical diagnoses. More and more research is emerging that substantiates the link between the mental state of the patient and propensity for recovery from illness or injury. The will to live is a very powerful thing and can often mean the difference between life and death. On the other hand, if an individual is despondent and lacks the will to survive, they will be much more susceptible to succumbing to an early and many times painful demise. A wise man once said that if you want to know what your mind was like in the past, just look at your body now. And if you want to know what your body will look like in the future, just look at your mind now.

Deepak Chopra wrote in <u>Ageless Body, Timeless Mind</u>: "We program our consciousness to a set span of aging, and our biology responds to that programming."

"I do not think seventy years is the time of a man or woman, nor that seventy millions of years is the time of man or woman, nor that years will ever stop the existence of me, or anyone else."

-Walt Whitman

Leaves of Grass

"Reality is merely an illusion albeit a very persistent one."

THINK OUTSIDE THE BOX
OR GO DOWN WITH THE SHIP

Comedian Stephen Colbert of the cable TV show "The Colbert Report" coined the word **truthiness** on Oct. 17, 2005. Truthiness, which was the Merriam- Webster word of the year in 2006, is defined as: 'Truth that comes from the gut, not books", and "The quality of preferring concepts or facts one wishes to be true, rather than concepts or facts that really are true."

Colbert suggested that truthiness is a characteristic of less intelligent or less thoughtful people because one does not find truthiness in a book. The social scientist Jay Stuart Snelson calls the resistance to changing one's paradigm "ideological immunity". Snelson noted that ideological immunity is actually found in more intelligent people. "Educated, intelligent, and successful adults rarely change their most fundamental presuppositions".

Regardless of basic intelligence, we become engrained at a very early age with a fundamental imprint of life that guides many of our perceptions later in life.
It would appear that those with higher intelligence can lose their objectivity in critical thinking. Sometimes Ego is our worst enemy.

It's easy to be skeptical or even cynical of data that falls outside of the box that we all create from our life experiences. This box, however, while protecting us from harm in some respects, can severely limit us in others. It's better to remain ignorant than to know so much that isn't so.

"Cognitive dissonance" is a term, much like "truthiness", that reflects the limits that our ego imposes upon us. We tend to view the world through defense mechanisms which can be propagated by fear of the unknown, unsubstantiated dogma, and/or unfettered ego. Information is meaningless and can't be comprehended unless we can put in it the context of what we have already learned. So, what if what we initially learned was wrong? Then, every subsequent piece of data is filtered through an inaccurate prism and usually leads to further misinterpretations. One can see how such views of reality can lead to much discord and controversy among individuals, religions and nations. How else could terrorists blatantly murder innocent people, all the while reveling in their accomplishments as the work of their god?

Imagine a three-year-old repeatedly watching drug commercials on television. He is likely to grow up believing that pharmaceuticals are a normal part of life. He doesn't know any better and at that age believes that whatever adults tell him must be true.

Some people believe they are so smart that no one can possibly know something they don't know. Quite possibly their perspective of how the world works is influenced by the business world they live in, where they see greed and profit motives controlling behavior. They can become quite jaded and cynical. This peculiar phenomenon is very common in overweight males who have achieved "success" in the business world, quite possibly in ways that they are none too proud of. These people don't know what they don't know and for one reason or another can't make that leap out of their little protective box. When faced with a health crisis they consider only what they are familiar with even when that approach is unsuccessful (or they ignore the crisis entirely). They literally choose to go down with the ship. One third of American adult males would not go to the doctor if they experienced shortness of breath, chest pains, or symptoms of a heart attack. While that mind-set may be baffling to some, it is perfectly understandable to those that are stuck in that paradigm.

"The cure for loneliness is solitude. Solitude can be defined as learning that we are not alone when we are alone, thereby achieving a conscious relationship with ourselves."

CONVICTIONS ARE MORE DANGEROUS ENEMIES OF TRUTH THAN LIES.

Friedrich Nietzsche

We need to view the human body as the precious gift that it is rather than taking it for granted. If someone repeatedly abuses or neglects their body in spite of being aware of the health consequences of such behavior, then they are deliberately committing suicide. They need to look at their motivations for such behavior.

"We can spend decades climbing the ladder only to realize too late that we have placed it against the wrong wall."
        Joseph Campbell

"We prize something called "success", yet become all the more miserable for having achieved it."

"Holding anger and resentment inside you is like drinking poison and hoping the other person dies."

WHAT ARE WE REALLY MADE OF?

Nature knows how it works; we don't, at least not yet. If/when we discover the theoretical and elusive Higg's boson, then some of nature's deepest secrets may at last be revealed; until then, we just don't know. The Standard Model will remain an unproven enigma until that time. Scientists are still finding things that they don't understand, but are rapidly closing in on some answers.

Dig deep inside the atom and you find tiny particles held together by invisible forces in a sea of empty space. Dig even further and we discover that everything is made up of tiny packets of energy born in cosmic furnaces. This energy that cools down, gets dragged through a mysterious force called the Higgs and clumps together to form all the things we call matter is itself an enigma.

It has an evil twin called antimatter; but most of that has long since disappeared. In the early universe, matter particles outnumbered antimatter particles by one part in a billion. Without that tiny, inexplicable discrepancy, matter would not exist at all and our very existence as well as that of all the planets and galaxies would be impossible.

As we get close to re-creating the heat of the Big

Bang in our accelerators, we get closer to understanding how and why all things happened; well, maybe not why. Perhaps, someday, not long from now, we'll finally solve the last remaining riddles of matter and fully comprehend the inner workings of creation. There still, however, is much work to do as answering one fundamental question often leads to several more. As a matter of fact, nature is really asking the questions and we are pretty much going along for the ride; but, oh what a ride it is.

"Life is not a problem to be solved but a reality to be experienced."

NATURE IS NOT ONLY STRANGER THAN WE THINK,

NATURE IS STRANGER THAN WE CAN THINK.

WHY WE THINK LIKE WE DO

Life experiences that affect us emotionally are amplified through the seat of emotion and memory stimulus portion of the brain called the limbic system, which is the gateway to higher cognition centers in the brain. The memory of the experience is relayed from the hypothalamus-amygdala-hippocampus complex to processing and memory centers for interpretation and storage. The brainstem to limbic system to neocortex pathway has been dubbed the heartbeat to heartstrings to heartless pathway. The volume of sensory data filtered through the brain is staggering.

Question: How many potential combinations of neuronal connections are possible in the average human brain?

    A. As many as there are elementary particles (atoms) in a golf ball.

    B. As many as there are elementary particles in the entire planet earth.

    C. As many as there are elementary particles our galaxy.

D. As many as there are elementary particles in the known universe.

The answer is at the bottom of this page.

The key to long-term retention of information or experiences relates strongly to your degree of emotional investment. Students learn more in classes that they enjoy than in classes they perceive as boring. My wife can remember mind-boggling details of vacations that we have taken over the years that leave me shaking my head in disbelief. I can remember certain unpleasant childhood experiences from as young as two or three years of age. Most people of my generation can remember details of where they were and what they were doing when they learned that JFK was shot in 1963.

The way we think as adults is influenced in a tremendous way by our life's experiences and our emotional interpretations of those experiences. We all need to be cognizant of the overwhelming effect we can have on small children as they perceive the world through strong emotional pathways while still lacking the capacity for sophisticated rational thought. Many adult dysfunctional behaviors can be traced to subliminal emotional input that has skewed their moralities and rational decision-making abilities. People can literally suffer from arrested development due to childhood emotional blocks. Sometimes they remain stuck in a certain place their entire lives.

Answer: D

"As we acquire more knowledge things do not become more comprehensible but more mysterious."

REASON-LOGIC-COMMON SENSE

God made man in His own image. As such God made man perfect in his design and function. How could it be any other way? He also made rules that would govern the function and order of the universe (and Nature). Then, he gave man a very special gift- **FREE WILL**. Man would always be governed by the Laws of Nature: Cause and Effect, Action and Reaction; but he would be free to choose to obey or disobey these Laws at his own discretion. **It is this free will that enabled man to make every decision that put him right where he is today.**

Gradually, man began to place himself above Nature by inventing an existence he believed to be above the rest of life. In his arrogance he considered himself immune to Natural Laws. He discovered stimulation and learned how to circumvent Nature's Laws to exact greater performance from his body. He lacked the foresight to realize that Nature's Laws were being violated and what is stimulated eventually becomes exhausted.

The cells of the body do not reason; they do, however, possess consciousness. They each have specific functions and only do as instructed by the nervous or endocrine system. If a cell does the right thing at the wrong time, it's due to faulty internal communications or interference through stimulation. The body does not make mistakes. Although we may not possess the necessary wisdom to understand, **everything the body does is for a reason.** Everybody response is appropriate for the environment we provide it in an attempt to maintain homeostasis. It will also sacrifice a part of itself to save the whole. That's where chronic disease comes from. The body tries to do the best it with the circumstances and environment we provide it and operates under a system of priorities. **We need to look at disease with appreciation and amazement.** Disease is the body's attempt to stay alive.

The present state of your health is a direct result of your lifestyle; your lifestyle is a result of your habits; your habits are a result of your preferences; and your preferences are a result of your beliefs. If you wish to change a condition that is a result of your lifestyle, habits and preferences, you must be willing to change your beliefs.

We must learn to use **REASON, LOGIC, and COMMON SENSE** to understand how the body really works. We must leave ego, arrogance, greed and corruption by the wayside if we are to solve the mysteries of life. We must come to realize that there are certain levels of consciousness and awareness where disease does not exist. Learn to accept the truth, ever if it flies in the face of conventional thinking and the way that you were taught. Remember, there is subjective reality and then **there is the way that things really are.**

*"The most comprehensible thing about universe
is that it is incomprehensible."*

*It's what you learn after
you know it all that counts!*